Vegan Gluten-fr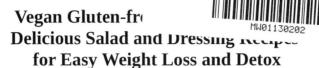
Delicious Salad and Dressing Recipes
for Easy Weight Loss and Detox

by **Vesela Tabakova**
Text copyright(c)2015 Vesela Tabakova

Table Of Contents

Vegan Gluten-free Salads and Dressings for Easy Weight Loss and Detox

Being healthy doesn't have to mean overhauling your entire lifestyle. Sometimes all it takes is a few simple changes in your diet. Eating a vegan gluten-free salad every day can have an enormous effect on your overall health and mood. Vegan gluten-free salads are ideal not only for a number of health conditions, but are also perfect if you just want to lose weight without starving and getting bored with your diet.

In a world where food is full of obscure artificial additives and flavorings, there is a simple and easy way to cook gluten-free and vegan food. So much of the food you already love is naturally gluten-free and, therefore, the safest way to follow a vegan gluten-free diet is to cook at home and to stick primarily to fresh unprocessed ingredients.

If you want to eat really healthy salads with whole food ingredients, it is best to make them yourself. It's really not that difficult to prepare your salads at home with fresh vegetables, herbs, and legumes, as well as other naturally gluten-free foods such as quinoa or buckwheat. It may sound difficult at first, but you will soon realize you can throw together a healthy salad in the same amount of time you'd need to order a takeout. Here are some quick and easy-to-make homemade vegan gluten-free salad recipes to get you started.

Roasted Leek, Watercress and Sweet Potato Salad

Serves 5

Ingredients:

1 lb sweet potato, unpeeled, cut into 1 inch pieces

3-4 leeks, trimmed and cut into 1 inch slices

a handful of baby spinach leaves

1 cup watercress, rinsed, patted dry and separated from roots

1 tbsp dried mint

2 tbsp olive oil

2 tbsp lemon juice

Directions:

Preheat the oven to 350 F. Line a baking tray with baking paper and place the sweet potato and leeks on it. Drizzle with olive oil and sprinkle with mint. Toss to coat. Roast for 20 minutes or until tender.

Place roasted vegetables, baby spinach and watercress in a salad bowl and stir. Sprinkle with lemon juice and serve.

Mediterranean Avocado Salad with Olives

Serves 5

Ingredients:

1 avocado, peeled, halved and cut into cubes

1 cup grape tomatoes

3-4 radishes, sliced

2 tbsp drained capers, rinsed

1 cucumber, quartered and sliced

a handful of rocket leaves

½ cup green olives, pitted, halved

½ cup black olives, pitted, sliced

7-8 fresh basil leaves, torn

2 tbsp olive oil

2 tbsp red wine vinegar

salt and pepper, to taste

Directions:

Place avocado, cucumber, tomatoes, radishes, rocket, olives, capers and basil in a large salad bowl.

Toss to combine then sprinkle with vinegar and olive oil. Season with salt and pepper, toss again and serve.

Avocado, Sweet Corn and Cucumber Salad

Serves 5

Ingredients:

2 avocados, peeled, halved and sliced

2-3 green onions, finely cut

1 cucumber, halved, sliced

1/2 cup cooked corn kernels

for the dressing:

2 tbsp olive oil

3 tbsp lemon juice

1 tbsp gluten free mustard

1/2 cup finely cut dill leaves

salt and pepper, to taste

Directions:

Combine avocado, cucumber, corn and green onions in a deep salad bowl.

Whisk olive oil, lemon juice, dill and mustard until smooth, then drizzle over the salad. Season with salt and pepper to taste, toss to combine and serve.

Artichoke and Bean Salad with Lemon Mint Dressing

Serves 5

Ingredients:

1 can white beans, drained

2/3 cup podded broad beans

4 marinated artichoke hearts, quartered

2/3 cup diced green bell pepper

for the dressing:

3 tbsp olive oil

3 tbsp lemon juice

1 tsp dried mint

5-6 fresh mint leaves, very finely cut

salt and pepper, to taste

Boil the broad beans in unsalted water for 3-4 minutes or until tender. Drain and hold under running cold water for a few minutes. Combine with the canned beans, bell peppers and quartered marinated artichoke hearts in a deep salad bowl.

In a small bowl, mix olive oil, lemon juice, dried mint and fresh mint. Whisk until smooth. Add in salt and pepper and pour over salad. Toss gently to combine and serve.

Artichoke and Mushroom Salad

Serves: 4-5

Ingredients:

1 oz can artichoke hearts, drained, cut quartered

7-8 white button mushrooms, chopped

1 red pepper, chopped

1/3 cup chopped black olives

1 tbsp capers

3 tbsp lemon juice

2 tbsp olive oil

salt and pepper, to taste

Directions:

Place the artichokes and mushrooms in a large salad bowl and stir to mix well. Add in olives, capers and red pepper and toss to combine.

In a small bowl, whisk the lemon juice and olive oil until smooth. Pour over the salad, toss and serve.

Superfood Salad

Serves 4

Ingredients:

7 oz cauliflower, cut into florets

7 oz baby Brussels sprouts, trimmed

7 oz broccoli, cut into florets

1/2 cup chopped leeks

for the dressing:

2 tbsp lemon juice

2 tbsp olive oil

1/2 tsp ginger powder

1/2 cup parsley leaves, very finely cut

Directions:

Cook cauliflower, broccoli and Brussels sprouts in a steamer basket over boiling water for 10 minutes or until just tender. Refresh under cold water for a minute and set aside in a deep salad bowl.

Whisk the lemon juice, olive oil and ginger powder in a small bowl. Add in salt and pepper to taste; pour over the salad. Top with parsley and serve.

Apple and Radicchio Salad

Serves 4-5

Ingredients:

1 radicchio, trimmed, finely shredded

2 apples, quartered and thinly sliced

a handful of rocket leaves

4-5 spring onions, chopped

½ cup walnuts, toasted

1 tbsp gluten free mustard

1 tbsp lemon juice or balsamic vinegar

3-4 tbsp olive oil

a little sea salt

Directions:

Prepare the dressing by combining mustard, lemon juice and olive oil.

Place walnuts on a baking tray and bake in a preheated to 400 F oven for 3-4 minutes, or until browned.

Mix radicchio, rocket, apples, onions and walnuts in a large salad bowl. Add the dressing; add sea salt, toss to combine and serve.

Apple, Celery and Walnut Salad

Serves 4

Ingredients:

3 large apples, quartered, cores removed, thinly sliced

1 celery rib, thinly sliced

½ cup walnuts, chopped

1 red onion, thinly sliced

2 tbsp raisins

1/4 cup sunflower seeds

3 tbsp apple cider vinegar

2 tbsp olive oil

salt and black pepper, to taste

Directions:

Mix vinegar, olive oil, salt and pepper in a small bowl. Whisk until well combined.

Place apples, celery, onion, walnuts, raisins and sunflower seeds in a bigger salad bowl. Drizzle with dressing, toss and serve.

Fresh Greens Salad

Serves 6-7

Ingredients:

1 head red leaf lettuce, rinsed, dried and chopped

1 head green leaf lettuce, rinsed, dried and chopped

1 head endive, rinsed, dried and chopped

1 cup frisee lettuce leaves, rinsed, dried and chopped

3-4 fresh basil leaves, chopped

3-4 fresh mint leaves, chopped

2-3 spring onions, chopped

1 tbsp chia seeds

4 tbsp olive oil

3-4 tbsp lemon juice

1 tsp sugar

salt, to taste

Directions:

Place the red and green leaf lettuce, frisee lettuce, endive, onions, basil and mint into a large salad bowl and toss lightly to combine.

Prepare the dressing from lemon juice, olive oil and sugar and pour it over the salad. Sprinkle with chia seeds and season with salt to taste.

Simple Beet Salad

Serves 4

Ingredients:

2-3 small beets, peeled

3-4 green onions, cut

3 cloves garlic, minced

2 tbsp red wine vinegar

2-3 tbsp sunflower oil

salt to taste

Directions:

Place the beats in a steam basket set over a pot of boiling water. Steam for about 12-15 minutes, or until tender. Leave to cool.

Grate the beets and put them in a salad bowl. Add the crushed garlic cloves, the finely cut green onions and mix well. Season with salt, vinegar and sunflower oil.

Beet Salad with Spinach and Walnuts

Serves 4

Ingredients:

3 medium beets, steamed and diced

1/2 bag baby spinach leaves

1 red onion, sliced

1/2 cup walnuts, halved and toasted

for the dressing:

1 garlic clove, crushed

2 tbsp lemon juice

2 tbsp olive oil

4-5 fresh mint leaves, chopped

½ tsp salt

Directions:

Place the beats in a steam basket set over a pot of boiling water. Steam for about 12-15 minutes, or until tender. Leave to cool for 5-6 minutes, then peel and dice the beets. Place the spinach leaves in a large salad bowl. Add in the beets, onion and walnuts.

In a smaller bowl, combine the oil, lemon juice, garlic and mint. Whisk and drizzle over the salad.

Beet Salad with Coconut Yogurt

Serves 4

Ingredients:

4 medium beets, steamed and cubed

1 cup coconut yogurt

2 garlic cloves, crushed

1/2 tsp dried mint

½ tsp salt

Directions:

Wash the beets and steam them over boiling water for 25-30 minutes, or until cooked through.

Peel and cut the beets in small cubes then place them in a deep salad bowl. Whisk the coconut yogurt with garlic, mint, and salt. Pour over the beets and toss to combine. Serve cold.

Pickled Beet and Lentil Salad

Serves 6

Ingredients:

1 can brown lentils, drained and rinsed

1 can pickled beets, drained and cut in cubes

5 oz baby rocket leaves

¼ cup walnuts, toasted and roughly chopped

4-5 green onions, chopped

1 garlic clove, crushed

3 tbsp olive oil

2 tbsp lemon juice

salt and black pepper, to taste

Directions:

Heat olive oil in a frying pan and gently sauté green onions for 1-2 minutes or until softened. Add in garlic and lentils. Cook, for 2 minutes the add in beets and cook for 2-3 minutes more.

Combine baby rocket, walnuts and lentil mixture in a large salad bowl. Sprinkle with lemon juice, toss gently to combine and serve.

Beet and Bean Sprout Salad

Serves 4-5

Ingredients:

5-6 beet greens, finely sliced

2 tomatoes, sliced

1 cup bean sprouts, washed

3 tbsp pumpkin seeds

1 tbsp grated lemon rind

2 garlic cloves, crushed

4 tbsp lemon juice

3 tbsp olive oil

1 tsp salt

Directions:

In a large bowl, toss together beet greens, bean sprouts, tomatoes and pumpkin seeds.

Combine oil and lemon juice with lemon rind, salt and garlic and pour over the salad. Serve chilled.

Roasted Vegetable Salad

Serves 4

Ingredients:

2 tomatoes, halved

1 medium zucchini, quartered

1 eggplant, ends trimmed, quartered

2 large red pepper, halved, deseeded, cut into strips

2-3 white mushrooms, halved

1 onion, quartered

1 tsp garlic powder

2 tbsp olive oil

for the dressing:

1 tbsp lemon juice

1 tbsp apple cider vinegar

2 tbsp olive oil

1 tsp sumac

5 tbsp crushed walnuts, to serve

Directions:

Whisk olive oil, lemon juice, vinegar and sumac in a bowl.

Preheat oven to 500 F. Place the zucchini, eggplant, peppers, onion, mushrooms and tomatoes on a lined baking sheet. Sprinkle with olive oil, season with salt, pepper and sumac and roast until golden, about 25 minutes. Divide in 4-5 plates, top with crushed walnuts, drizzle with the dressing and serve.

Warm Quinoa Salad

Serves 6

Ingredients:

1 cup quinoa

½ cup green beans, frozen

½ cup sweet corn, frozen

½ cup carrots, diced

½ cup black olives, pitted and halved

2-3 garlic cloves, crushed

2 tbsp fresh dill, finely cut

3 tbsp lemon juice

2 tbsp olive oil

Directions:

Wash quinoa with lots of water. Strain it and cook it according to package directions. When ready, set aside in a large salad bowl and fluff with a fork.

Heat olive oil in a large saucepan over medium heat. Stew green beans, sweet corn, olives and carrots until vegetables are tender. Add this mixture to quinoa and stir to combine.

In a smaller bowl, combine lemon juice, dill and garlic and pour over the warm salad. Add salt and black pepper to taste and serve.

Quinoa and Black Bean Salad

Serves 6

Ingredients:

1 cup quinoa

1 cup black beans, cooked, rinsed and drained

½ cup sweet corn, cooked

1 red bell pepper, deseeded and chopped

4-5 spring onions, chopped

2 garlic cloves, crushed

1 tbsp dry mint

3 tbsp lemon juice

½ tsp salt

4 tbsp olive oil

Directions:

Rinse quinoa in a fine sieve under cold running water until the water runs clear. Put quinoa in a pot with two cups of water. Bring to a boil, then reduce heat, cover and simmer for fifteen minutes or until water is absorbed and quinoa is tender. Fluff with a fork and set aside to cool.

Put beans, corn, bell pepper, spring onions and garlic in a salad bowl and toss to combine. Add quinoa and toss well again.

In a smaller bowl whisk together lemon juice, salt and olive oil and drizzle over the salad. Toss well and serve.

Roasted Vegetable Quinoa Salad

Serves 6

Ingredients:

2 zucchinis, cut into bite sized pieces

1 eggplant, peeled and cut into bite sized pieces

3 roasted red peppers, peeled cut into bite sized pieces

4-5 small white mushrooms, whole

1 cup quinoa

½ cup olive oil

2 tbsp apple cider vinegar

1 tsp summer savory

salt and pepper, to taste

Directions:

Toss the zucchinis, mushrooms and eggplant in half the olive oil, salt and black pepper. Place on a baking sheet in a single layer and bake in a preheated 350 F oven for 30 minutes flipping once.

Wash well, strain, and cook quinoa following package directions.

Prepare the dressing from the remaining olive oil, apple cider vinegar, summer savory, salt and black pepper. In a big bowl combine quinoa, roasted zucchinis, eggplant, mushrooms and roasted red peppers. Toss the dressing into the salad.

Quinoa with Oven Roasted Tomatoes and Pesto

Serves 6

Ingredients :

1 cup quinoa

2 cups water

1 cup cherry tomatoes, for roasting

½ cup cherry tomatoes, fresh

1 avocado, cut into chunks

½ cup black olives, pitted

for the pesto

2 cloves garlic, chopped

½ tsp salt

½ cup walnuts, toasted

1 cup basil leaves

1 tbsp lemon juice

4-6 tbsp olive oil

1 tsp summer savory

2 tbsp water (optional)

Directions:

Preheat the oven to 350 F and line a baking sheet with foil or baking paper. Wash and dry a cup of cherry tomatoes, arrange them on the baking sheet, drizzle with olive oil and savory and toss to coat well. Bake the tomatoes for about twenty minutes, flipping once, until they are brown. Sprinkle with salt.

Rinse quinoa very well in a fine mesh strainer under running water; set aside to drain. Place two cups of water and quinoa in a large saucepan over medium-high heat. Bring to the boil, then reduce heat to low. Simmer for fifteen minutes. Set quinoa aside, covered, for ten minutes and fluff with a fork.

Make the homemade pesto by placing garlic, walnuts and ½ teaspoon of salt in a food processor. Add basil and lemon juice and blend in batches until smooth. Add oil, one tablespoon at a time, processing in between, until the pesto is light and creamy. Taste for salt and add more if you like.

In a large mixing bowl, gently mix the quinoa with the tomatoes, avocado and olives. Spoon in the pesto and toss to distribute it evenly.

Cucumber Quinoa Salad

Serves 6

Ingredients:

1 cup quinoa

2 cups water

1 large cucumber, diced

½ cup black olives, pitted

2 tbsp lemon juice

2 tbsp olive oil

1 bunch fresh dill, finely cut

Directions:

Wash quinoa very well in a fine mesh strainer under running water and set aside to drain. Place quinoa and two cups of cold water in a saucepan over high heat and bring to the boil. Reduce heat to low and simmer for fifteen minutes. Set aside, covered, for ten minutes, then transfer to a large bowl.

Add the finely cut dill, diced cucumber and olives and toss to combine.

Prepare a dressing from the lemon juice, olive oil, salt and pepper. Add it to the salad and toss to combine.

Fresh Vegetable Quinoa Salad

Serves 6

Ingredients:

1 cup quinoa

2 cups water

a bunch of spring onions, chopped

2 green peppers, chopped

½ cup black olives, pitted and chopped

2 tomatoes, diced

1 cup sunflower seeds

3 tbsp olive oil

4 tbsp fresh lemon juice

1 tbsp dried mint

Directions:

Prepare the dressing by combining olive oil, lemon juice and dried mint in a small bowl and mixing it well. Place the dressing in the refrigerator until ready to use.

Wash well and cook quinoa according to package directions. When it is ready leave it aside for ten minutes, then transfer it to a large bowl.

Add the diced peppers, finely cut spring onions, olives and diced tomatoes, stirring until mixed well. Stir the dressing (it will have separated by this point) and add it to the salad, tossing to evenly coat. Add salt and pepper to taste and sprinkle with sunflower seeds.

Warm Mushroom Quinoa Salad

Serves 4-5

Ingredients:

1 cup quinoa

2 cups gluten free vegetable broth

1 tbsp sunflower oil

2-3 spring onions, chopped

2 garlic cloves, chopped

10 white mushrooms, sliced

1-2 springs of fresh rosemary

½ cup dried tomatoes, chopped

2 tbsp olive oil

salt and freshly ground black pepper

½ bunch fresh parsley, finely cut

Directions:

Wash well the quinoa in plenty of cold water, strain it and put it in a saucepan. Add vegetable broth and bring to the boil. Lower heat and simmer for ten minutes until the broth is absorbed.

Heat oil in a frying pan and sauté onions for 2-3 minutes. Add garlic and sauté for another minute. Add sliced mushrooms and season with salt and pepper. Add the rosemary and cook the mushrooms until soft.

Combine quinoa with mushrooms and dried tomatoes. Serve sprinkled with fresh parsley.

Quinoa Tabbouleh

Serves 6

Ingredients:

1 cup quinoa

2 cups water

2 cups parsley leaves, finely cut

2 tomatoes, chopped

3 tbsp olive oil

2 garlic cloves, minced

6-7 spring onions, chopped

2-3 tbsp fresh mint leaves, chopped

juice of two lemons

salt and black pepper, to taste

Directions:

Rinse quinoa very well in a fine mesh strainer under running water; set aside to drain. Place water and quinoa in a large saucepan over medium-high heat. Bring to the boil, then reduce heat to low. Simmer for 15 minutes. Set aside, covered, for 10 minutes.

In a large bowl, mix together the finely cut parsley, tomatoes, olive oil, garlic, spring onions and mint. Stir in the already chilled quinoa and season to taste with salt, pepper, and lemon juice.

Quinoa and Asparagus Salad

Serves 6

Ingredients:

1 cup quinoa

2 cups water

10-11 asparagus stalks, woody ends trimmed, cut

2 bell peppers, deseeded, chopped

¼ cup sunflower seeds

4 spring onions, chopped

2 tbsp fresh parsley, finely cut

2 tbsp lemon juice

1 tsp sugar

2 tbsp olive oil

1 tsp paprika

Directions:

Rinse quinoa very well in a fine mesh strainer under running water; set aside to drain. Place water and quinoa in a large saucepan over medium-high heat. Bring to the boil then reduce heat to low. Simmer for 15 minutes or until just tender. Set aside, covered, for 10 minutes.

Preheat an electric grill or grill pan and cook the asparagus for 2-3 minutes, or until tender crisp. Combine the asparagus, bell pepper, sunflower seeds, spring onions and parsley with the quinoa.

Whisk the lemon juice, sugar, oil and paprika in a small bowl until well combined. Add the dressing to the quinoa mixture. Season with black pepper and toss to combine.

Warm Cauliflower and Quinoa Salad

Serves 4

Ingredients:

1 small cauliflower, cut into bite sized pieces

1 cup quinoa

2 cups water

1 tbsp paprika

salt, to taste

½ bunch spring onions, finely cut

5-6 tbsp olive oil

Directions:

Preheat oven to 350 F. Cut the cauliflower into bite sized pieces and place it in a roasting dish. Toss in olive oil, salt and paprika and roast, stirring occasionally until golden on the edges and soft.

Wash quinoa well and place in a medium saucepan with two cups of water. Simmer for 15 minutes then set aside for 3-4 minutes. Serve quinoa topped with cauliflower and sprinkled with spring onions.

Quinoa, Zucchini and Carrot Salad

Serves 6

Ingredients:

1 cup quinoa

2 cups water

2 big carrots, sliced lengthwise into thin ribbons

1 zucchini, sliced lengthwise into thin ribbons

1 big cucumber, sliced lengthwise into thin ribbons

for the dressing:

2 garlic cloves, minced

2 tbsp orange juice

1 tbsp apple cider vinegar

2 tbsp olive oil

Directions:

Rinse the quinoa very well in a fine mesh strainer under running water; set aside to drain. Place water and quinoa in a large saucepan over medium-high heat. Bring to the boil then reduce heat to low. Simmer for 15 minutes or until just tender. Set aside, covered for 10 minutes.

Peel lengthwise the carrots and zucchini into thin ribbons. Steam them for 3-4 minutes. Peel the cucumber into ribbons too.

Prepare a dressing by mixing the orange juice, vinegar, olive oil and minced garlic.

Serve quinoa on each plate and arrange some of the vegetable stripes over it. Top with 2-3 tablespoons of the dressing.

Spicy Buckwheat Vegetable Salad

Serves 4-5

Ingredients:

1 cup buckwheat groats

2 cups gluten-free vegetable broth

2 tomatoes, diced

½ cup spring onions, chopped

½ cup parsley leaves, finely chopped

½ cup fresh mint leaves, very finely chopped

½ yellow bell pepper, chopped

1 cucumber, peeled and cut into 1/4-inch cubes

½ cup cooked or canned brown lentils, drained

1/4 cup freshly squeezed lemon juice

1 tsp gluten-free hot pepper sauce

salt, to taste

Directions:

Heat a large, dry saucepan and toast the buckwheat for about three minutes. Boil the vegetable broth and add it carefully to the buckwheat. Cover, reduce heat, and simmer until buckwheat is tender and all liquid is absorbed. Remove from heat, fluff with a fork and set aside to cool.

Chop all vegetables and add them together with the lentils to the buckwheat. Mix the lemon juice and remaining ingredients well and drizzle over the buckwheat mixture. Stir well to distribute the dressing evenly.

Mediterranean Buckwheat Salad

Serves 4-5

Ingredients:

1 cup buckwheat groats

1 3/4 cups water

1 small red onion, finely chopped

½ cucumber, diced

1 cup cherry tomatoes, halved

1 yellow bell pepper, chopped

a bunch of parsley, finely cut

1 preserved lemon, finely chopped

1 cup chickpeas, cooked or canned, drained

juice of half lemon

1 tsp dried basil

2 tbsp olive oil

Directions:

Heat a large dry saucepan and toast the buckwheat for about three minutes. Boil the water and add it carefully to the buckwheat. Cover, reduce heat and simmer until buckwheat is tender and all liquid is absorbed (5-7 minutes). Remove from heat, fluff with a fork and set aside to cool.

Mix the buckwheat with the chopped onion, bell pepper, cucumber, cherry tomatoes, parsley, preserved lemon and chickpeas in a salad bowl.

Whisk the lemon juice with olive oil and basil, season with salt and pepper to taste, pour over the salad and stir.

Buckwheat Salad with Asparagus and Roasted Peppers

Serves 4-5

Ingredients:

1 cup buckwheat groats

1 3/4 cups gluten-free vegetable broth

½ lb asparagus, trimmed and cut into 1 inch pieces

4 roasted red bell peppers, diced

1 tomato, diced

2-3 spring onions, finely chopped

2 garlic cloves, crushed

1 tbsp red wine vinegar

3 tbsp olive oil

½ cup fresh parsley leaves, finely cut

Directions:

Heat a large dry saucepan and toast the buckwheat for about three minutes. Boil the vegetable broth and add it carefully to the buckwheat. Cover, reduce heat and simmer until buckwheat is tender and all liquid is absorbed (5-7 minutes). Remove from heat, fluff with a fork and set aside to cool.

Cook the asparagus in a steamer basket or colander, 2-3 minutes until tender. Transfer it in a large salad bowl along with the roasted peppers and diced tomato. Add in the spring onions, garlic, red wine vinegar, salt, pepper and olive oil. Stir to combine. Add the buckwheat to the vegetable mixture. Sprinkle with parsley and toss the salad gently. Serve at room temperature.

Roasted Broccoli Buckwheat Salad

Serves 4-5

Ingredients:

1 cup buckwheat groats

1 3/4 cups water

1 head of broccoli, cut into small pieces

1 lb asparagus, trimmed and cut into 1 inch pieces

½ cup roasted cashews

for the dressing:

5-4 cup basil leaves, minced

½ cup olive oil

2 garlic cloves, crushed

Directions:

Arrange vegetables on a baking sheet and drizzle with olive oil. Roast in a preheated to 350 F oven for about fifteen minutes or until tender.

Heat a large, dry saucepan and toast the buckwheat for about three minutes, or until it releases a nutty aroma. Boil the water and add it carefully to the buckwheat. Cover, reduce heat and simmer until buckwheat is tender and all liquid is absorbed (5-7 minutes). Remove from heat, fluff with a fork and set aside to cool.

Prepare the dressing by blending basil leaves, olive oil, garlic, and salt.

Toss vegetables, buckwheat and dressing together in a salad bowl. Add in cashews and serve.

Light Superfood Salad

Serves 4

Ingredients:

1 cup mixed green salad leaves

2 cups watercress, rinsed, patted dry and separated from roots

4-5 green onions, chopped

1 avocado, peeled and cubed

10 radishes, sliced

10 green olives, pitted and halved

for the dressing:

2 tbsp lemon juice

2 tbsp apple cider vinegar

2 tbsp olive oil

1 tbsp gluten free mustard

1/2 tsp dried mint

Directions:

Combine all ingredients in a large salad bowl.

In a medium bowl or cup, whisk lemon juice, vinegar, olive oil, mint and mustard until smooth. Pour over salad, toss, and serve.

Baby Spinach Salad

Serves 4

Ingredients:

1 bag baby spinach, washed and dried

1 red bell pepper, cut in slices

1 cup cherry tomatoes, cut in halves

1 red onion, finely chopped

1 cup black olives, pitted

for the dressing:

1 tsp dried oregano

1 large garlic clove

3 tbsp red wine vinegar

4 tbsp olive oil

salt and freshly ground black pepper, to taste

Directions:

Prepare the dressing by blending the garlic and the oregano with the olive oil and vinegar in a food processor.

<

Place the spinach leaves in a large salad bowl and toss with the dressing. Add the rest of the ingredients and give everything a toss again. Season to taste with black pepper and salt.

Spinach and Asparagus Salad

Serves 4

Ingredients:

2 cups asparagus, woody ends trimmed, cut into 3 inch lengths

1 bag baby spinach

7-8 cherry tomatoes, halved

2-3 green onions, cut

1 cup cashews, coarsely chopped

for the dressing:

2 tbsp olive oil

1 tbsp white wine vinegar

1 garlic clove, crushed

salt and black pepper, to taste

Directions:

Boil the asparagus in a medium saucepan for 3-4 minutes until bright green and tender crisp. rinse under running cold water; drain well.

Whisk the dressing ingredients in a small bowl until smooth. Season with salt and pepper to taste.

Combine the asparagus, spinach, tomatoes and onions in a large serving bowl. Drizzle with the dressing, toss to combine, top with cashews and serve.

Roasted Pumpkin and Spinach Salad

Serves 4

Ingredients:

3 cups pumpkin, deseeded, peeled and cut into wedges

1/2 bag baby spinach leaves

1/2 cup canned chickpeas, drained

1/3 cup toasted hazelnuts, coarsely chopped

1 small red onion, thinly sliced

2 tbsp olive oil

2 tbsp maple syrup

for the dressing:

2 tbsp olive oil

2 tbsp lemon juice

1 garlic clove, crushed

Directions:

Preheat oven to 350 F. Line a baking tray with baking paper. Place pumpkin, maple syrup and olive oil in a bowl. Toss to combine. Season with salt and pepper and toss again. Place pumpkin, in a single layer, on prepared tray. Bake, turning once, for 20-30 minutes or until the pumpkin is tender. Set aside for to cool.

In a small bowl, whisk the dressing ingredients until smooth. Season with salt and pepper to taste.

Place the pumpkin, spinach, chickpeas, onion and hazelnuts in a large salad bowl. Drizzle with the dressing, toss, and serve.

Spinach Stem Salad

Serves 2-3

Ingredients:

about 9-10 spinach stems

water to boil the stems

2 garlic cloves, crushed

lemon juice or red wine vinegar, to taste

3-4 tbsp olive oil

salt, to taste

Directions:

Trim the stems so that they remain whole and wash them very well. Steam stems in a steamer over boiling water for 2-3 minutes, until wilted but not too soft.

Place the spinach stems on a plate and sprinkle with crushed garlic, olive oil, lemon juice or vinegar, and salt to taste.

Spinach and Green Bean Salad

Serves 5

Ingredients:

10 oz green beans, halved diagonally

1 bag baby spinach leaves

2/3 cup almonds, roasted

1 cup grape tomatoes

4-5 green onions, chopped

for the dressing:

1 tbsp gluten free mustard

1 tbsp olive oil

1 tbsp apple cider vinegar

2 garlic cloves, crushed

1 tsp dried mint

Directions:

Cook beans in a large saucepan of boiling salted water for 1-2 minutes. Rinse under cold water, drain, and pat dry.

Combine all dressing ingredients in a small glass bowl and whisk until smooth.

Place beans, spinach, almonds, grape tomatoes and onions in a salad bowl and toss to combine. Pour the dressing over and serve.

Green Bean and Radicchio Salad with Green Olive Dressing

Serves: 4

Ingredients:

1 lb trimmed green beans, cut to 2-3 inch long pieces

1 radicchio, outer leaves removed, washed, dried

1 small red onion, finely cut

1 cup cherry tomatoes, halved

green olive dressing

1/2 cup green olives, pitted

1/2 cup olive oil

2 garlic cloves, chopped

black pepper and salt, to taste

Directions:

Roughly tear the radicchio leaves and place on a large serving platter.

Steam or boil green beans for about 3-4 minutes until crisp-tender. In a colander, wash with cold water to stop cooking, then pat dry and arrange over the radicchio leaves.

Add in red onion and cherry tomatoes.

To make the green olive dressing, place the olives in a food processor and blend until finely chopped. Gradually add the oil and process until a smooth paste is formed. Taste and season with salt and pepper then spoon over salad and serve.

Easy Green Bean Salad

Serves 6

Ingredients:

2 cups canned green beans, drained

1 small onion, sliced

4 garlic cloves, crushed

3-4 fresh mint leaves, chopped

a bunch of fresh dill, finely chopped

3 tbsp olive oil

1 tbsp apple cider vinegar

salt and pepper, to taste

Directions:

Put the green beans in a medium bowl and mix with onion, mint and dill.

In a smaller bowl, stir olive oil, vinegar, garlic, salt and pepper until smooth. Pour over the green bean mixture and serve.

Three Bean Salad

Serves: 4

Ingredients:

½ cup canned white beans, drained and rinsed

1 lb trimmed green beans, cut to 2 inch long pieces

½ cup canned chickpeas, drained and rinsed

1 red pepper, thinly sliced

1 yellow pepper, thinly sliced

1/2 red onion, thinly sliced

for the dressing:

1 tbsp died basil leaves

2 tbsp olive oil

1 tsp garlic powder

1 tbsp red wine vinegar

salt, to taste

Directions:

Steam green beans for about 3-4 minutes until crisp-tender. rinse with cold water, pat dry and place in a salad bowl. Mix in the chickpeas, white beans, onions and peppers.

In a small bowl, whisk together the vinegar, olive oil, basil and salt. Pour over the salad, toss gently to combine and serve.

Greek Chickpea Salad

Serves 4

Ingredients:

1 cup canned chickpeas, drained and rinsed

1 spring onion, thinly sliced

1 small cucumber, diced

2 green peppers, diced

2 tomatoes, diced

2 tbsp chopped fresh parsley

1 tsp capers, drained and rinsed

juice of ½ a lemon

2 tsp olive oil

1 tsp balsamic vinegar

salt and pepper, to taste

a pinch of dried oregano

Directions:

In a medium bowl, toss together the chickpeas, spring onion, cucumber, green peppers, tomatoes, parsley, capers and lemon juice.

In a smaller bowl, stir together the remaining ingredients and pour over the chickpea salad. Toss well to coat and allow to marinate, stirring occasionally, for at least 1 hour before serving.

Spring Salad

Serves 4

Ingredients:

1 green lettuce, washed and drained

1 cucumber, sliced

a bunch of radishes, sliced

a bunch of spring onions, finely cut

juice of half lemon or 2 tbsp of white wine vinegar

3 tbsp olive oil

salt to taste

Directions:

Cut the lettuce into thin strips. Slice the cucumber and the radishes as thinly as possible and chop the spring onions.

Mix all the salad ingredients in a large bowl, add the lemon juice and olive oil and season with salt to taste.

Cabbage and Turnip Salad

Serves 4

Ingredients:

7 oz fresh white cabbage, shredded

7 oz carrots, shredded

7 oz white turnips, shredded

½ a bunch of parsley

2 tbsp white wine vinegar

3 tbsp sunflower oil

salt, to taste

Directions:

Combine cabbage, carrots and turnip in a large bowl and mix well. Add salt,vinegar and oil. Stir and sprinkle with parsley.

Red Cabbage Salad

Serves 6

Ingredients:

1 small head red cabbage, cored and chopped

1 bunch of fresh dill, finely cut

3 tbsp sunflower oil

3 tbsp red wine vinegar

1 tsp sugar

2 tsp salt

black pepper to taste

Directions:

In a small bowl, mix the oil, red wine vinegar, sugar and black pepper.

Place the cabbage in a larger glass bowl. Sprinkle the salt on top and crunch it with your hands to soften.

Pour the dressing over the cabbage and toss to coat. Sprinkle the salad with dill, cover it with foil and leave it in the refrigerator for half an hour before serving.

Okra Salad

Serves 4

Ingredients:

1.2 lb young okras

1 lemon

½ bunch parsley, chopped

2 tomatoes, sliced

for the dressing:

3 tbsp sunflower oil

½ tsp black pepper

salt, to taste

Directions:

Trim okras, then wash and cook them in salted water until tender. Drain and set aside to cool.

In a small bowl mix well the lemon juice and sunflower oil, salt and black pepper.

Arrange okra and tomatoes in a bowl then pour over the dressing and sprinkle with chopped parsley.

Cucumber Salad

Serves 4

Ingredients:

2 medium cucumbers, peeled and sliced

a bunch of fresh dill, finely cut

2 cloves garlic, minced

3 tbsp white wine vinegar

5 tbsp olive oil

salt, to taste

Directions:

Cut the cucumbers in rings and put them in a salad bowl.

Add the finely cut dill, the pressed garlic, and season with salt, vinegar and oil. Toss to combine and serve cold.

Simple Broccoli Salad

Serves 4

Ingredients:

14 oz fresh broccoli, cut into florets

3-4 fresh onions, finely cut

1/3 cup raisins

1/3 cup sunflower seeds

for the dressing:

1 garlic clove, crushed

1/4 cup orange juice

3 tbsp olive oil

Directions:

Combine broccoli, onions, raisins, and sunflower seeds in a medium salad bowl.

In a smaller bowl whisk the orange juice, garlic and olive oil until blended. Pour over the broccoli mixture and toss to coat.

Carrot and Apple Salad

Serves 4

Ingredients:

4 carrots, shredded

1 apple, peeled, cored and shredded

2 garlic cloves, crushed

2 tbsp lemon juice

salt and pepper, to taste

Directions:

In a salad bowl, combine the shredded carrots, apple, lemon juice, garlic, salt and pepper. Toss and chill before serving.

Roasted Eggplant and Pepper Relish

Serves 4

Ingredients:

2 medium eggplants

2 red or green bell peppers

2 tomatoes

3 cloves garlic, crushed

fresh parsley

1-2 tbsp red wine vinegar

olive oil, as needed

salt, pepper

Directions:

Wash and dry the vegetables. Prick the skin off the eggplants. Bake the eggplants, tomatoes and peppers in a preheated oven at 480 F, for about 40 minutes, or until the skins are well burnt. Take out of the oven and leave in a covered container for about 10 minutes.

Peel the skins off and drain well the extra juices. De-seed the peppers.

Cut all the vegetables into small pieces. Add the garlic and blend everything well with a fork or in a food processor. Add the olive oil, vinegar and salt to taste. Stir again. Serve cold and sprinkled with parsley.

White Bean Salad

Serves 4-5

Ingredients:

1 cup white beans

1 onion, cut

3 tbsp white wine vinegar

1 bunch of fresh parsley

salt and black pepper

Directions:

Wash the beans and soak them in cold water to swell overnight. Cook in the same water with the peeled onion. When tender, drain and put into a deeper bowl. Remove the onion.

Mix well oil, vinegar, salt and pepper. Pour over the still warm beans, leave to cool about 30-40 minutes. Chop the onion and the parsley, add to the beans, mix and leave to cool for at least 40 minutes. Serve cold.

Roasted Peppers with Garlic and Parsley

Serves 4-6

Ingredients:

2.25 lb red and green bell peppers

½ cup sunflower oil

1/3 cup white wine vinegar

3-4 cloves garlic, chopped

a bunch of fresh parsley

salt and pepper, to taste

Directions:

Grill the peppers or roast them in the oven at 480 F until the skins are a little burnt. Place the roasted peppers in a brown paper bag or a lidded container and leave covered for about 10 minutes. This makes it easier to peel them.

Peel the skins and remove the seeds. Cut the peppers into 1 in strips lengthwise and layer them in a bowl. Mix together the oil, vinegar, salt and pepper, chopped garlic and chopped parsley leaves. Pour over the peppers. Cover the roasted peppers and chill for an hour.

FREE BONUS RECIPES: 20 Easy Vegan, Gluten-Free, Superfood Smoothies for Better Health and Natural Weight Loss

Mango and Asparagus Smoothie

Serves: 2

Prep time: 5 min

Ingredients:

1 frozen banana, chopped

1 cup water or green tea

1 mango, peeled and chopped

½ cup raw asparagus, chopped

1 lime, juiced

1 tsp sesame seeds

Directions:

Combine ingredients in a blender and purée until smooth. Enjoy!

Pineapple and Asparagus Smoothie

Serves: 2

Prep time: 5 min

Ingredients:

2-3 ice cubes

1 cup apple juice

1 pear, cut

½ cup raw asparagus, chopped

½ cup pineapple, chopped

2-3 mint leaves

Directions:

Combine ingredients in a blender and purée until smooth. Enjoy!

Fennel and Kale Smoothie

Serves: 2

Prep time: 5 min

Ingredients:

1-2 ice cubes

1 cup coconut water

1 cup fennel

2-3 kale leaves

2-3 fresh figs

2 limes, juiced

Directions:

Combine ingredients in a blender and purée until smooth. Enjoy!

Kids' Favorite Kale Smoothie

Serves: 2

Prep time: 5 min

Ingredients:

2-3 ice cubes

1½ cup apple juice

1 small apple, cut

½ cup pineapple chunks

½ cucumber, cut

3 leaves kale

Directions:

Combine ingredients in a blender and purée until smooth. Enjoy!

Kids' Favorite Spinach Smoothie

Serves: 2

Prep time: 5 min

Ingredients:

1 frozen banana

1 cup orange juice

1 apple, cut

1 cup baby spinach

1 tsp vanilla extract

Directions:

Combine ingredients in a blender and purée until smooth. Enjoy!

Paleo Mojito Smoothie

Serves: 2

Prep time: 5 min

Ingredients:

1 cup ice

1 cup coconut water, milk or plain water

1 big pear, chopped

2-3 limes, juiced, or peeled and cut

20-25 leaves fresh mint

3 dates, pitted

Directions:

Juice the limes or peel and cut them and combine with the other ingredients in a blender. Process until smooth. Enjoy!

Winter Greens Smoothie

Serves: 2

Prep time: 5 min

Ingredients:

2 broccoli florets, frozen

1½ cup coconut water

½ banana

½ cup pineapple

1 cup fresh spinach

2 kale leaves

Directions:

Combine ingredients in blender and blend until smooth. Enjoy!

Delicious Kale Smoothie

Serves: 2

Prep time: 5 min

Ingredients:

2-3 ice cubes

1½ cup apple juice

3-4 kale leaves

1 apple, cut

1 cup strawberries

½ tsp cloves

Directions:

Combine ingredients in blender and purée until smooth.

Cherry Smoothie

Serves: 2

Prep time: 5 min

Ingredients:

2-3 ice cubes

1½ cup almond or coconut milk

1½ cup pitted and frozen cherries

½ avocado

1 tsp cinnamon

1 tsp chia seeds

Directions :

Combine all ingredients into a blender and process until smooth. Enjoy!

Banana and Coconut Smoothie

Serves: 2

Prep time: 5 min

Ingredients:

1 frozen banana, chopped

1½ cup coconut water

2-3 small broccoli florets

1 tbsp coconut butter

Directions :

Add all ingredients into a blender and blend until the smoothie turns into an even and smooth consistency. Enjoy!

Avocado and Pineapple Smoothie

Serves: 2

Prep time: 5 min

Ingredients:

3-4 ice cubes

1½ cup coconut water

½ avocado

2 cups diced pineapple

Directions:

Combine all ingredients in a blender, and blend until smooth. Enjoy!

Carrot and Mango Smoothie

Serves: 2

Prep time: 5 min

Ingredients:

1 cup frozen mango chunks

1 cup carrot juice

½ cup orange juice

1 carrot, chopped

1 tsp chia seeds

1 tsp grated ginger

Directions:

Combine all ingredients in a blender, and blend until smooth. Enjoy!

Strawberry and Coconut Smoothie

Serves: 2

Prep time: 5 min

Ingredients:

3-4 ice cubes

1½ cup coconut milk

2 cups fresh strawberries

1 tsp chia seeds

Directions:

Place all ingredients in a blender and purée until smooth. Enjoy!

Beautiful Skin Smoothie

Serves: 2

Prep time: 5 min

Ingredients:

1 cup frozen strawberries

1½ cup green tea

1 peach, chopped

½ avocado

5-6 raw almonds

1 tsp coconut oil

Directions:

Place all ingredients in a blender and purée until smooth. Enjoy!

Kiwi and Pear Smoothie

Serves: 2

Prep time: 5 min

Ingredients:

1 frozen banana, chopped

3 oranges, juiced

2 kiwi, peeled and halved

1 pear, chopped

1 tbsp coconut butter

Directions:

Juice oranges and combine all ingredients in a blender then blend until smooth. Enjoy!

Tropical Smoothie

Serves: 2

Prep time: 5 min

Ingredients:

2-3 ice cubes

1½ cup coconut water

½ avocado

1 mango, peeled, diced

1 cup pineapple, chopped

2-3 dates, pitted

Directions:

Place all ingredients in a blender and purée until smooth. Enjoy!

Melon Smoothie

Serves: 2

Prep time: 5 min

Ingredients:

1 frozen banana, chopped

1-2 frozen broccoli florets

1 cup coconut water

½ honeydew melon, cut in pieces

1 tsp chia seeds

Directions:

Combine all ingredients in a blender, and blend until smooth.

Healthy Skin Smoothie

Serves: 2

Prep time: 5 min

Ingredients:

1 cup frozen berries

1 cup almond milk

½ avocado

1 pear

1 tbsp ground pumpkin seeds

1 tsp vanilla extract

Directions :

Put all ingredients in a blender and blend until smooth. Enjoy!

Paleo Dessert Smoothie

Serves: 2

Prep time: 5 min

Ingredients:

1 frozen banana

1 cup coconut water

1 cup raspberries

2 apricots, chopped

1 tbsp almond butter

Directions:

Put all ingredients into blender. Blend until smooth. Enjoy!

Easy Superfood Smoothie

Serves: 2

Prep time: 5 min

Ingredients:

3-4 ice cubes

1½ cup green tea

1 pear, chopped

½ cup blueberries

½ cup blackberries

1 tbsp almond butter

Directions :

Place all ingredients in a blender and blend for until even. Enjoy!

About the Author

Vesela lives in Bulgaria with her family of six (including the Jack Russell Terrier). Her passion is going green in everyday life and she loves to prepare homemade cosmetic and beauty products for all her family and friends.

Vesela has been publishing her cookbooks for over a year now. If you want to see other healthy family recipes that she has published, together with some natural beauty books, you can check out her <u>Author Page</u> on Amazon.

Made in the USA
Coppell, TX
08 November 2021

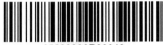